OVER 50
OVERWEIGHT
and

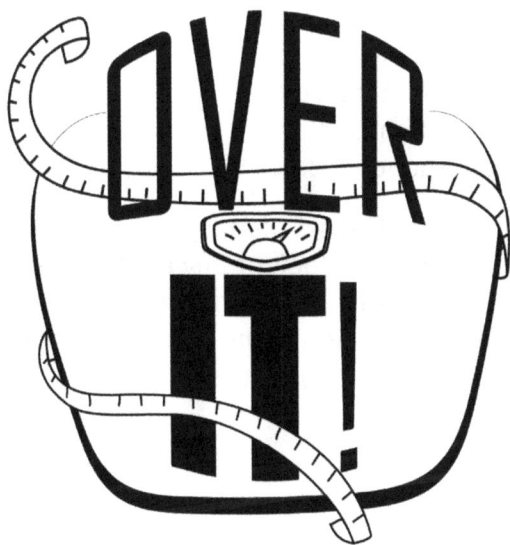

OVER IT!

MELINDA DICKEY

OVER 50, OVERWEIGHT AND OVER IT!
Melinda Dickey
© 2021 Melinda Dickey
ISBN: 978-0-578-32432-6

Cover Design: April Robinson
Text Design: Lisa Simpson
www.simpsonproductions.net

Contents

Contents

Introduction

So, I had a great Christmas vacation with my family in the mountains. There were 10 of us in a beautiful cabin in Georgia and we ate goood! I had been thinking for several months that I needed to do something about my weight, but just couldn't seem to find the motivation. Maybe it was the family pictures, where I was getting too big to hide behind people. Or, maybe it was the fact that I couldn't walk or hike with the rest of them, without getting winded. But, somewhere on that trip I decided I had enough and I was OVER it!

I waited to start the process until January 2. I wanted to enjoy every second of the holidays before I started. So, on January 2, I started my journey. I needed to lose 57 lbs. My aim was to lose 5 lbs a month. I weighed 207 and was a size 20. It is now December and I have lost 57 lbs! I weigh 150 lbs for the first time in 20 years. From a size 20 to a size 12! I have more energy and feel so much better! I wanted to help others get healthy as well.

I would share my progress on Facebook and loved the fact that my friends rejoiced with me and cheered me on. As I lost more and more weight so many of them asked me how. What are you doing?

I share my experience with you. I hope this helps. I am by no means an expert and of course, everyone is different. And, you know, check with your doctor before starting anything, etc. But, every doctor will tell you 60 lbs overweight is not healthy. Some of you have less and some of you have more to lose, but if you don't start somewhere, a year from now you will either be heavier, or the same. I wanted to be 60 lbs lighter, 60 lbs healthier, 60 lbs better.

Remember if you always do what you've always done you are always going to be just where you are. Or, if you do nothing different, next year at this time, you may be heavier than you are now. And, you will be less healthy. It's time for change.

I have tried many times over the years and just about every diet plan out there. I tease and say "I lost a hundred pounds last year", but it was the same 10 pounds over and over again! I had to reach a point to decide, once and for all I'm done.

I was over 50 and overweight and finally OVER it! …..

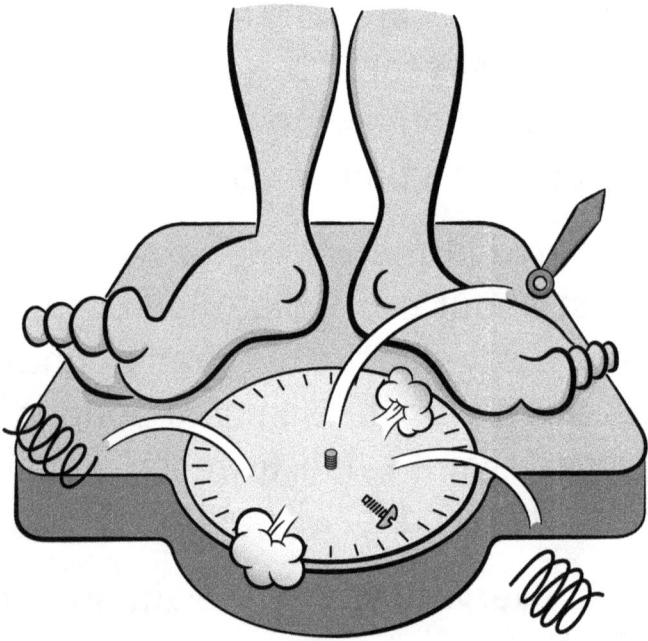

Chapter 1

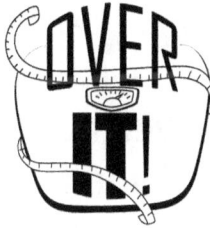

The Motivation —
The Decision

This may not be the largest chapter in this book, but it has to be the most important. You have to be able to find the motivation to keep on keeping on! Whatever it takes.

The biggest motivation for me is the fear of growing old and being feeble. My dad had a saying "The only alternative to growing old is dying young". At 63 years old, I realize more than ever that growing old is inevitable. Growing old is not a choice, but how you do it is!

We have all seen the people in the grocery stores that can't get around unless they have a scooter cart. I don't want my future to be walkers, wheelchairs, and portable oxygen. And, yes weight isn't all of it, but it is a big part of it. If you think 60 lbs doesn't make a difference, try carrying around two 30 lb bowling balls for a day and see if you can move better without them.

You know how much obesity affects your overall health. Risk of diabetes, heart problems, stroke and even cancer increase greatly with obesity. In this time of covid, remember that one of the comorbidity issues is obesity. Your immune system is weaker when you are overweight.

I knew a 90 something year old lady who would climb up on her roof to sweep the leaves off. Now, I don't care how healthy I am, I can't see me ever climbing up on the roof to do anything! But, I would like to know at age 90 something that I could if I wanted to.

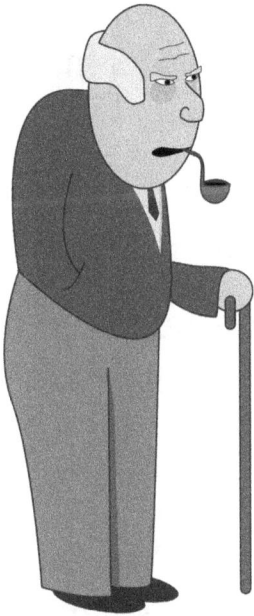

How do you want your 60s or 70s or even 80s to be? I just saw on FB where my friends from highschool went zip-lining at age 64. I will probably never go zip-lining. I will probably never again go downhill skiing or scuba diving. But, I would like to be healthy enough that just getting in the boat wouldn't tucker me out!

Do you want to be able to roll around on the floor with your grand babies? Or your great-grand babies? (By the way, I may have been able to roll around on the floor, but I wouldn't have been able to get up without help).

Do you want to be able to walk or hike without having to stop and catch your breath? Or climb the stairs without passing out?

I will never be able to run a marathon (nor do I want to), but I am walking 3 miles a day and believe it or not I enjoy it.

Would you like to get dressed and look in the mirror and feel better about yourself?

I realize my days of turning heads and wolf whistles are over. I will never again look good in a bikini. But, I do look a lot better in my new skinny clothes!

One day not too long ago, we had cleaned out our cash jar (rainy day savings) for a special offering. My niece saw this and jokingly commented on all the small bills. She told me when we see bills like that we just assume you have started stripping. She asked, "Have one of you guys become a stripper?" I replied, "No, these days they pay me to keep my clothes on...and the pay is really good"!

It's not about looks … It's about health. Certainly, I look better in my skinny clothes, and I have loads more self-confidence. But the best result is my overall better health.

I was heading toward diabetes and a stroke. I was on blood pressure medication and I had to be on round-the-clock anti-inflammatories to ease arthritis pain. I am now off of all blood pressure medications, my doctor says my triglycerides are good, and I can't remember the last time my joints hurt so bad I needed an anti-inflammatory. My cholesterol is better and my energy is through the roof!

The motivation for losing weight has to be for your good health. It has to be about feeling good and enjoying life. It has to be about having more energy and being able to do more. And, it has to be long-term. There is no quick fix. No miracle cure. It is going to take work and determination. It is going to take grit, and perseverance. You didn't wake up one morning overweight. And, you won't be able to fix it overnight.

I was blessed with a great metabolism when I was younger. I never had a weight problem until I was in my mid-40's. But, oh my goodness as the hormones waned the weight gained. And, it became a battle. I could no longer eat like I used to. And, with each year I just gained more and more. I would crash diet. I've tried diet fads and diet pills. I eventually threw in the towel and just got heavier and heavier.

I once had a job selling flooring. I did quite well though the hours were brutal. One day I had an appointment at this huge house (mansion-like, 10 bedrooms and a pool house). I was still relatively new with this company and I was overwhelmed. I didn't think I could manage a quote for new flooring for the entire house. I called my manager and told him I needed help. He wasn't able to come help me, but he did quote an old

proverb. "How do you eat an elephant?"...
The answer is "one bite at a time". Just take
it one room at a time.

That's how we need to approach weight
loss. If we look at the enormity of the situ-
ation, we can easily be overwhelmed. Just
take it one month … 5 lbs at a time.

If you are reading this book, you are more
than likely over 50 and overweight. But, are
you over it?

It has to be a lifestyle, a life changing, life
altering decision, a course correction.

When my daughter was growing up,
we would have our "fun times" where she
just didn't want to do as she was told. But
she knew if I got to the point where I said
"Ethany, I am done!", it was time for her to
get up and do what I was asking her to do.
I had reached that point. I finally came to
that point with myself, my health, and my
weight. I am done! I am over it!

Here are a number of reasons to start .. and to start now!

1. I want to feel better about myself

2. I just want to feel better

3. I want to have more energy

4. I don't want another year to go by like this

5. I don't want a stroke

6. I don't want a heart attack

7. I don't want diabetes (or I want to better manage diabetes).

8. I'm sick and tired of being sick and tired

9. I want to be able to keep up with my grandkids

10. I'm tired of my clothes not fitting

11. I'm tired of shopping in the plus sizes

12. I don't want to be a burden to my family later in life.

13. I want to get healthy and STAY healthy

14. I want a stronger immune system

15. I don't want to have to hide when someone takes a photograph.

16. I want to climb in and out of cars without help.

17. I want to fit into a booth at a restaurant

18. I know losing weight will reduce my risk of getting cancer.

19. I want to sleep better

20. I want to be able to look back on the last 12 months and feel like I have accomplished something positive.

21. I don't want the joint pain that comes with the extra pounds.

22. I want to be able to touch my toes (or at the least, see my toes).

23.

24.

25.

I have intentionally left some blanks. You need to come up with your own reasons. Make a top 10 list of the most important reasons for you to do this and stick with it!

Make the list. Put it on your bathroom mirror. Read it aloud everyday! Especially when it gets hard and you feel like quitting.

I don't mean to imply that this will always be a white knuckle time and that every step of the way will be a battle. It gets easier and I have some good advice to help you get there. But it all comes down to a decision. A "come hell or high water" decision. No holds barred, no looking back. I will burn my bridges and my fat clothes decision!

I will talk more about the "how to" in the later chapters. But the "decision to" has to come from way down in your heart. I do have a question for you though. If not now, then when?

Top 10 Reasons to Lose Weight and Get Healthy

1. _____

2. _____

3. _____

4. _____

5. _____

6. _____

7. _____

8. _____

9. _____

10. _____

When will enough be enough?

If while reading this you have come up with half a dozen reasons to not try or not to start, then you may be over 50 and you may be overweight but you are not yet OVER it.

If you are ready. Here's a great way to start. Go ahead and finish reading the book, learn all the tips and then come back to this.

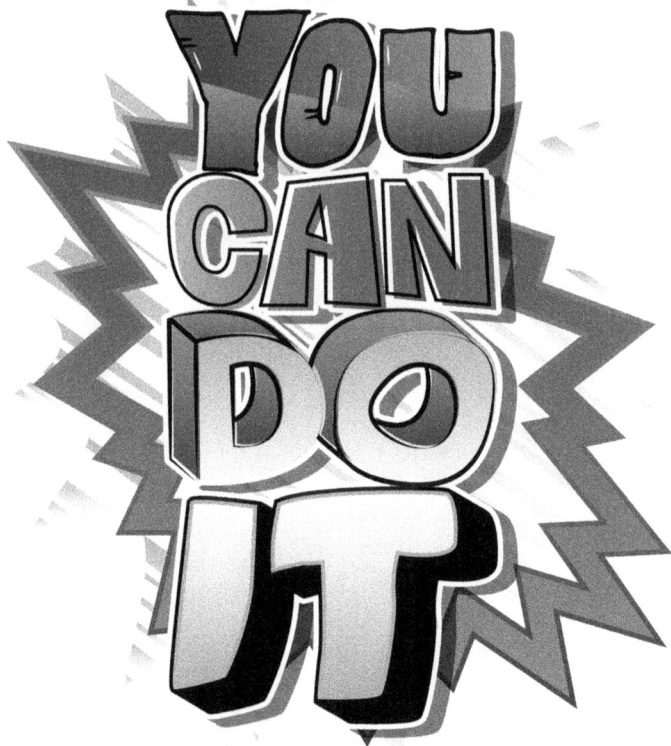

(Obviously, if you don't need to lose 60 lbs. You can adjust the months. But whatever it is ….start now!)

I also want to say that if you are reading this book, and you are not yet over 50 but you are overweight. You need to start now. I don't want to be the bearer of bad news, but, it will not get any easier. It will be so much more difficult. Start now! Go into your 50's a happier healthier you!

Print out or tear out the following. Fill it out. Put it on your fridge and stick to it.

Date: _____

I _____ am making the decision to change my life. I will start today. I will lose 5 lbs per month for the next year. By the end of this year ... I will be healthier, happier and 60 lbs lighter.

Signed,

_____

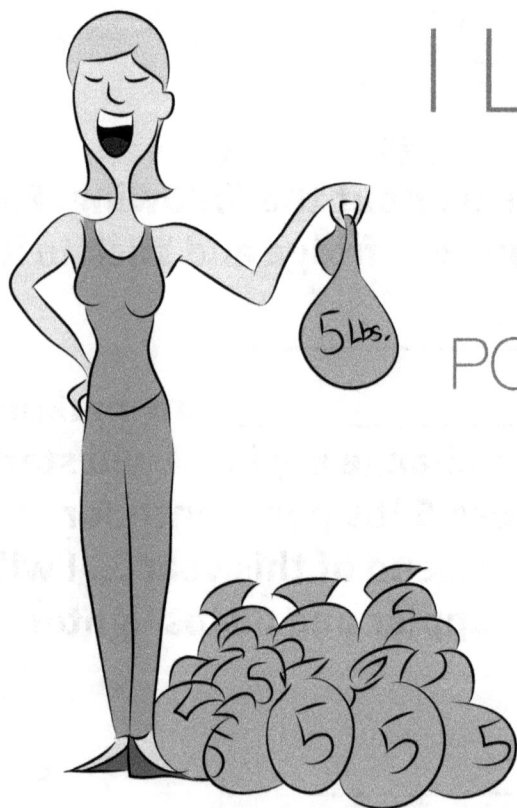

Chapter 2

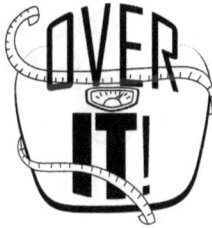

The Long Haul

There are many diets that promise quick results, but I have found that most of those are not sustainable and not healthy. The doctors tell us 4-6 lbs a month is much better than trying to lose too much too quickly. I keep seeing advertisements for pills that can help you lose 40 lbs in 20 days. There is no way that can be a healthy choice (even if it is possible). Your body isn't built that way. If you go into starvation mode, every part of your body will suffer. You may end up being skinnier, but you won't be healthier.

In this microwave, instant message, over-night delivery world, we want everything now! I know patience is a virtue and appar-ently I am not very virtuous. The absolute biggest reason that we fail when it comes to dieting and weight loss is we don't see the results quickly enough. I promise you if you start now, you will start to feel better and have more energy in just a month's time. You will be surprised at how it gets progres-sively better and better.

At 207 lbs I was overweight. I was 57 lbs heavier than I wanted to be. At 5'5" I was considered obese. I decided that I was going to lose 5 lbs a month and in one year's time I will have reached my goal weight. I would be 150 lbs.

You do the math. How much do you need to lose? Give yourself one year and see what a difference 60 lbs can make. If you need to lose more just keep going. If it takes 2 years wouldn't it be better to start now?

Here are some tips to keep you motivated.

Make small goals

Today, I ate well. Today, I exercised. Today I am on track. Maybe it's as simple as: Today I didn't overeat. Today, I didn't eat the whole pie. Today, I didn't eat the entire bag of chips. I am making changes and I am making progress.

Remember even if you take 3 steps forward and 2 steps backwards, you will eventually get there. It may take you a little longer... But keep heading in the right direction.

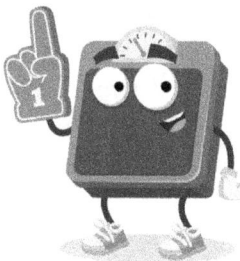

If you have a bad day, or even a bad week, get back up! Put on your big girl pants and start again.

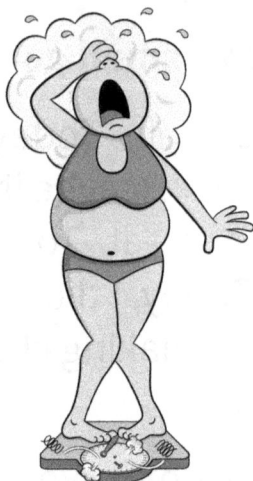

Try not to focus too much on the scale

Your weight can fluctuate a lot even in one day. I try to weigh in only twice a month. On the 15th to make sure that I'm still on track for the month, and on the 2nd (because I started on January 2).

Celebrate the victories

I started posting on facebook my progress and how much I had left to lose. It was great to have my friends celebrate each small goal with me and cheer me on.

Get a calendar mark off the days. Make a big poster to hang on your wall. 5 down and only 20 to go!! Celebrate the small victories and keep on track for the long haul.

Tell yourself, "you can do this!" Plan ahead for the celebration. Buy some smaller clothes and celebrate when you fit into them! I was so excited to finally fit into size 14 jeans.

Let your doctor know. It's fun to watch the blood work come back better each time!

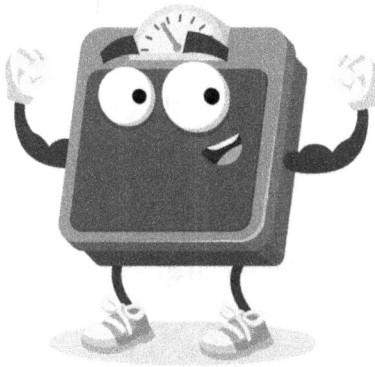

Surround yourself with cheerleaders

It helps to tell some people. Choose those you know love you and want the best for you. I chose FB, but also my close family and friends. They would always tell me how proud they were and encourage me. You can do it!

Accountability

Telling people also gave me a little accountability. It helped me to stay on track. I didn't want to embarrass myself by failure.

Keep a journal

It does help you to journal your day. Today, I did well. Today I stayed on track. Today I reached my goal for the month. Today I actually fit into those old jeans. This journaling will help you to see your progress. It may also help you to recognize some pitfalls. Keep a diary!

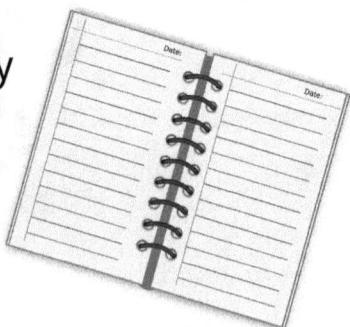

Get a money jar

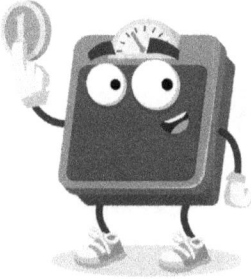

Get a money jar. Every day/week put in the money you would have spent on ice cream, candy bars, donuts, french fries or sodas. This can be your savings toward your new skinny wardrobe! Watch your savings grow as you shrink!

Sign up for a Walk-a-Thon

Find a charity walk, for a cause you like. Find a date 3 or 6 months out. This will help you to get in shape so you can complete the walk.

Get back up and keep going

We will talk more in future chapters about how to avoid pitfalls and to overcome the slip ups. But, the bottom line is get up, dust off and keep on going! What's the alternative? You don't want to give up now. You don't want to stop. And, you surely don't want to go back!

This is doable and you can do it!

Chapter 3

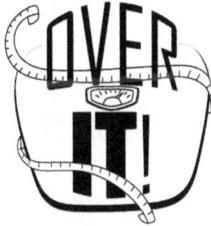

The Eating Part

The simplest way to understand dieting or losing weight is to understand that you must burn more calories than you consume. If you eat less and exercise more, simple physics will tell you — you will lose weight.

Unfortunately, especially if you are over 50, it's more difficult to burn off the excess calories. I have found that simple calorie counting diets don't work for me. For me it had to be more about the types of calories I was consuming rather than just the amount.

You have heard about low-carb diets. Years ago it was called the Atkins diet. The South Beach and the Keto Diet all work on the same basic concept. There is a reason why these diets work. It's all about your blood sugar level. It's about ketosis, metabolizing your fat cells for energy.

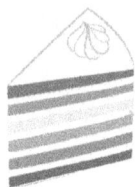

I will attempt to explain what happens in your body as you consume high sugar/high carbohydrate foods. I have taken an organic chemistry course, but I really cannot scientifically explain all of your metabolic reactions to foods. And, honestly, I don't fully comprehend it all.

I have read enough documentation to at least have a basic understanding of the process. I will do my best to explain it.

When you partake of high sugar/high carbohydrate foods, your blood sugar level will rise. In an attempt to regulate that sugar level your pancreas will get to work to lower that level. Your body will ask do I need this for energy now? If not, your body will store that excess sugar in your fat cells.

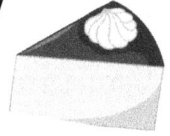

I recently saw a meme that said "Fat cells must have accepted Jesus as their savior as they seem to have eternal life and live forever."

I know your goal is not to store away more fat.

If you do not consume high sugar/high carbohydrate foods, when you need energy, your body has been designed to go to your fat cells to break them down for energy.

This is I'm sure over simplified. And, for type 1 diabetics it is a lot more complicated.

However, the reason why overweight people are so much more prone to type 2 diabetes is that we overwork our pancreas.

Our bodies were not designed to have to continue regulating this type of eating.

The other reason that the low-carb lifestyle menu works is that it effectively eliminates the cravings.

You know the cycle. You eat and then you crave. This has to do with your blood sugar levels. When your blood sugar spikes your body over-works to lower it. When your blood sugar lowers too much too quickly, you crave more food.

When you overeat and store more food as fat, you weigh more. You have less energy. You burn less fat. You eat more and you do less. It gets worse and worse.

That's why for me I couldn't lose weight on just the calorie counting alone. I would say I can eat a baked potato because it is only so many calories. But, it is a high-glycemic food that will spike your blood sugar and the cycle will continue.

You can search on the internet for a list of low-glycemic foods and that can help you to stay on track. Thankfully, the low-carb diet is fairly common and it is easy to find healthy choices in foods. There are many great recipes for low carb/keto friendly meals.

I have included a list of low-glycemic foods (foods that won't spike your blood sugar). And, with the help of the internet it's not difficult to look up.

There is another BIG reason to eliminate processed sugar from your diet. I took this quote directly off the internet.

"Studies have shown spikes in sugar intake suppress your immune system. When your immune system is compromised, you are more likely to get sick. If you eat lots of foods and beverages high in sugar or refined carbohydrates, which the body processes as sugar,

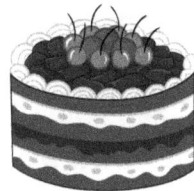

you may be reducing your body's ability to ward off disease."[1]

But the long and short of it is — your intake of sugar, breads, pastas and starches has to be drastically reduced.

Now I realize this is heartbreaking for most of you. And, you may require a day of mourning to overcome this cold hard fact. Take the day, cry and wail and eat your bonbons. And, if this is too much for you to bear, then again … You may be over 50 and you may be overweight, but you are not yet OVER it.

Sugar was my biggest downfall. (Though I have never met a potato I didn't like). I used to tell people that I was on a very strict "sugar-only" diet. I would start the morning with donuts and finish the day with ice cream.

I know where every McDonalds in the city is and I have been known to stop at 3 of

[1] *https://www.piedmont.org/living-better/foods-and-drinks-that-compromise-your-immune-system*

them in a half hour trip to get an ice cream. I love bagels and could eat 10 of them in a day covered with cream cheese.

I love chocolate. I remember hearing someone say that she kept a candy bar in the cupboard and when she had a sweet tooth, she would just take a bite and put it back. I never had that kind of willpower. If it was there, I would eat it. I would eat the entire bag of candy bars. I didn't trust myself with the Halloween candy. I have consumed huge bags of candy corn in a day. The chocolate covered eggs would be long gone before Easter. It was never a big mystery to me why I was overweight.

Thankfully, there are some great choices for sweet toothed people like me. I have found that some of the Atkins bars or their Endulge bars can get me through. I always feel like I need something sweet after a salty meal and these types of low carb snacks have met that need.

There are alternative sweeteners to sugar. I use an Equal packet in my coffee and if I have oatmeal I will use one on that as well. But, there are healthier alternatives. But, remember these artificial sweeteners are not good for you if you consume them in great quantities.

Believe it or not whipped cream is low on the glycemic index. I used it in my coffee. (The problem was I ended up using an entire can in my coffee). So, if you can keep it in stock without overdoing it, use whipped cream.

You will, however, be pleasantly surprised at how sweet other things become once you eliminate the refined sugars from your diet. I never ate fruits before, but I love them now. They are much sweeter to me now.

And, I promise you the overwhelming cravings will not be there if you "cleanse" yourself from the high-glycemic foods.

So, you may be thinking ...
What *CAN* I eat?

Well, you can eat all vegetables (except corn and cooked carrots). Meat, cheese, eggs and nuts will not spike your blood sugar. Fruits are good (except bananas and watermelon).

Sweet potatoes are low-glycemic. Oatmeal is also.

When it comes to breads, **all** breads are high-glycemic. However, your high-wheat, high bran breads are lower in glycemic value than your white breads.

The reason why white breads, cooked carrots and mashed potatoes are considered high-glycemic foods is that your body can digest them more quickly. These foods break-down way too easily into sugar.

Here's a trick ... if you absolutely have to have a piece of bread or a starchy food, balance it with some high protein food. It will help to stop your blood sugar from spiking too high.

You will also be able to see on the glycemic charts that some foods will surprise you and be lower on the charts than you would anticipate. For example potato chips are not as high on the chart as white bread. It's because the fat surrounding the potato chips doesn't allow your body to break them down as quickly.

Now that doesn't by any means imply that they are good for you. But if you are at a luncheon and have to choose between a sandwich and potato chips, take the sandwich, eat the inside (not the bread) and a handful of potato chips. Obviously, you can't eat the whole bag.

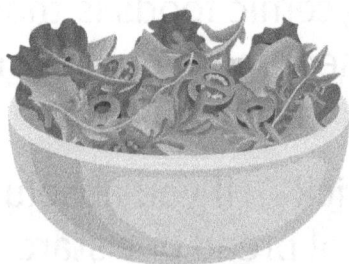

I eat lots of salads. I can order a Chef Salad from our local restaurant and it will last for two meals. If I'm in the mood I will cook a steak and a baked sweet potato and some green beans and I will be full.

I will have a hamburger with all the fixins with no bun. That's what I normally order when I'm at a restaurant. I also found a great recipe for cheeseburger soup complete with the pickles!

I suggest you carry a protein bar with you for emergencies.

I eat small meals throughout the day, and I keep snack foods available. Little smokies (sausages) work for a quick meal. Raw carrots, sliced cucumber and some grapes with a couple of slices of cheese will fill me up. Boil up some eggs in advance and leave them in the fridge. Have them with some ranch dressing.

A handful of almonds make a good snack. Be careful with the nuts however, they are still high calorie foods.

I do drink protein shakes. I like the Atkins shakes but there are a lot of different kinds to choose from. Watch the labels and look at the overall net carbs and the sugars.

My breakfast usually consists of a protein shake and a protein bar. However, occasionally I will have eggs and bacon and some sliced tomatoes. My point is there are lots of foods that can fill you up and help you to avoid the cravings. I don't go hungry.

I intentionally don't give you a planned menu to follow. You need to come up with your own based on your likes and dislikes. If you like to cook, there are thousands of low carb/keto friendly recipes out there.

Make a plan and stick to it. I eat less now than I did a year ago, because my stomach has shrunk. You don't have to go hungry, just choose the right foods.

Also notice, I am not giving you a calorie count to hit or even an overall number of carbs. Everyone is different. Your rate of metabolism is based partly on age, partly on muscle mass, partly on hormones and also partly on how you have trained your body over time.

However, if you are reading this book, more than likely you need to increase your metabolic rate. So, keep away from the carbs and burn off more than you consume. You will see how this works for you. If you aren't losing weight after a month, eat less and work out more. It really isn't rocket science.

I also have found that the calorie counting/ writing down everything you eat, type of diets, etc. aren't really designed to work for the rest of your life. I know you've heard this before, but to sustain weight loss over the long term, you are going to have to change your lifestyle.

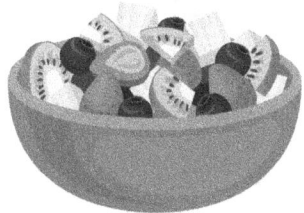

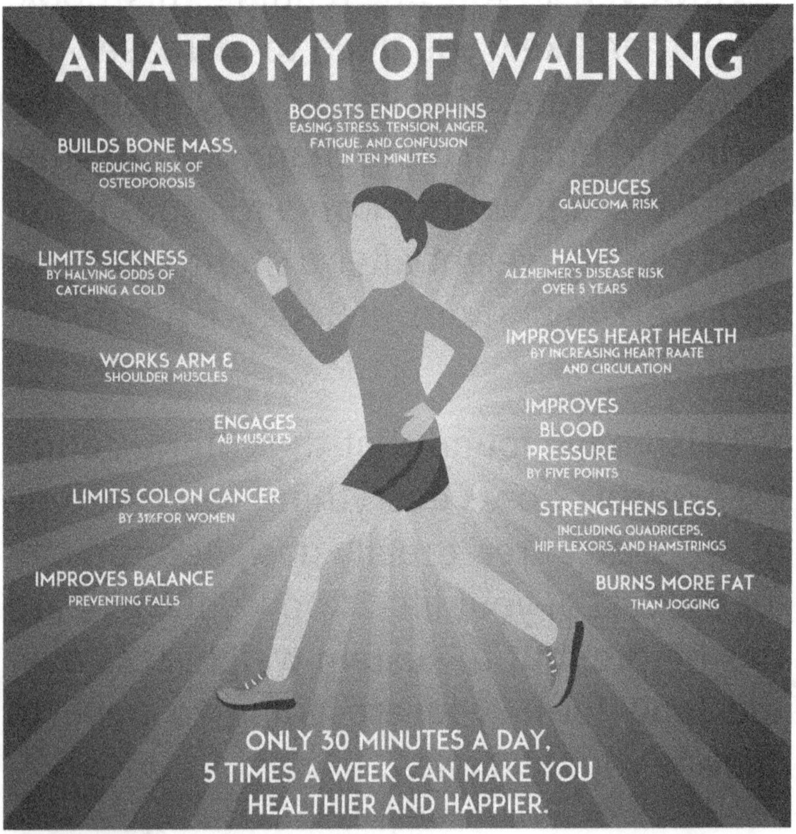
ANATOMY OF WALKING
BOOSTS ENDORPHINS
EASING STRESS, TENSION, ANGER, FATIGUE, AND CONFUSION IN TEN MINUTES
BUILDS BONE MASS,
REDUCING RISK OF OSTEOPOROSIS
REDUCES
GLAUCOMA RISK
LIMITS SICKNESS
BY HALVING ODDS OF CATCHING A COLD
HALVES
ALZHEIMER'S DISEASE RISK OVER 5 YEARS
IMPROVES HEART HEALTH
BY INCREASING HEART RAATE AND CIRCULATION
WORKS ARM &
SHOULDER MUSCLES
ENGAGES
AB MUSCLES
IMPROVES BLOOD PRESSURE
BY FIVE POINTS
LIMITS COLON CANCER
BY 31%FOR WOMEN
STRENGTHENS LEGS,
INCLUDING QUADRICEPS, HIP FLEXORS, AND HAMSTRINGS
IMPROVES BALANCE
PREVENTING FALLS
BURNS MORE FAT
THAN JOGGING
ONLY 30 MINUTES A DAY, 5 TIMES A WEEK CAN MAKE YOU HEALTHIER AND HAPPIER.

Chapter 4

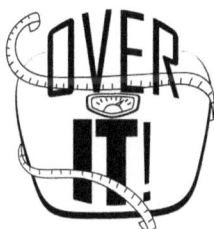

Get the move on

I promise you exercise is not a four letter word. Get moving! Your heart and your entire circulatory system will benefit from exercise. Your respiratory system will be stronger. Your weight will decrease and your energy will increase.

Walking

I have never been a runner. I've tried at different times and

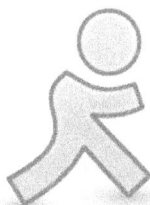

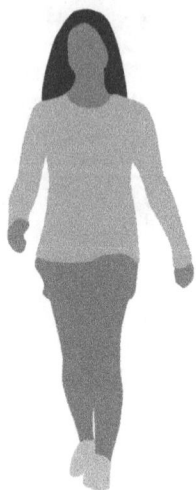

I realize you can burn calories more quickly with running. But, at 63 I found my joints couldn't handle it and I hated every minute of it. I needed something more low impact so I started walking.

Every phone has a step tracker or you can download an app. The step trackers that you can wear on your wrist are relatively inexpensive. I have a Samsung phone and I don't even need to start the app. It just detects me walking and keeps track of my steps. Start with small goals and build up every week. Don't try and start out with too much. Set your pace and try a little further and a little faster every day.

I started out walking just down the street and even that would tire me out and I was winded. Then eventually I was able to walk around the entire block. Then a whole mile. It took endurance and time to build up. I walk a lot faster now and farther than I did when I first started. When I started, I would walk with my husband, he would outpace me. Now I outpace him.

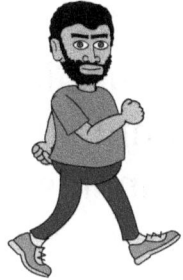

I have a treadmill, but I have found I don't enjoy it as much. Even if I watch a show while I am walking, I get bored too quickly. I have a route outside in my neighborhood that I walk and can see my progress.

Now, I live in Florida. Summertime in Florida is oh my goodness hot! Thankfully, I have a route that is mostly in the shade. The trick is to go early. I also have a portable, rechargeable fan that I bought on Amazon and I wear it around my neck. I am now up to 3 miles a day and I am able to keep a steady pace of around 3.5 miles/hour.

Most days I walk in my neighborhood. But on the weekends, we go on nature hikes. We live near a wilderness preserve and we will take the 3 mile loop around. I have an autistic son, he is 17 years old. He enjoys the walks. I encourage you to get your kids walking. Help them to develop good habits.

When I was a kid, we would leave the house in the morning and not come home until supper time. We were on our bikes, running, swimming, and moving all day long. Kids today, unfortunately, have a much more sedentary lifestyle. We have got to get our kids moving.

If you choose to walk outside, stay safe and stay hydrated.

I also realize that I am semi-retired and have a lot more time than someone who works full time. But, my mother had a saying … "You will always find the time to do what you really want to do."

You don't have to be outside to get your steps in. Walk around your house. Stay inside where it is air conditioned. Just get your steps in. Wake up 15 minutes early and walk around your house. Go to work early and walk around the parking lot. Take your lunch break and walk around the parking lot, or walk up and down the hallway inside. Get a headset and pace back and forth at your desk while you are on the phone.

Wherever you go, park out in the farthest spot in the parking lot and walk. When you go to the grocery store, park far away and walk. When you come back with your cart, don't just put it in the slot, walk it all the way back to the front of the store. Make a list of the groceries you need and do your shopping one item at a time even if the next item is all the way across the store. People may think you are crazy. But, eventually you will be crazy skinny! You can laugh all the way to the dress shop!

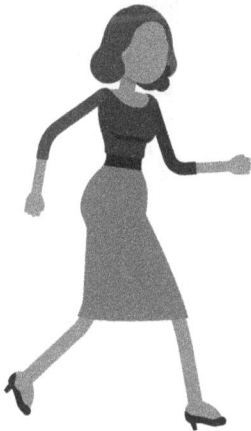

If there is a wait at the doctor's or dentist office. Don't just sit there. Ask if they can call you when you are next to be seen. Walk up and down the parking lot or up and down the outside hallway.

If you take your kids to the pool -- don't just sit there. Watch them, but walk around the pool. Or get in and do some water aerobics. Stay moving!

My mother-in-law had a group of ladies that used to walk around the mall, inside and air-conditioned. However, she did tell me they enjoyed the sitting and talking at the food court more than the walking.

If you take your kids to football/soccer or baseball practice, don't just sit there. Walk around the field, walk around the parking lot. My niece used to jog around the football field while her son was at practice.

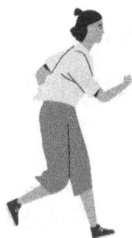

I keep my tennis shoes on after I come back from my walk. I find that when I'm just doing chores and walking around the house, I walk faster with my walking shoes on.

If you sweep or vacuum a room -- do it twice. You will get more steps in, expend more energy and your house will be cleaner for it.

Put your laundry away a little at a time so you have to keep walking back and forth to the laundry room.

If you have to wait in a car line for your kids, go early. If you are there before school lets out, and the cars aren't moving. Walk, walk, walk.

If you are flying somewhere, don't just sit at the gate. Walk around the gate area. If there's a wait at the restaurant and they give you the beeper/or text you when your table is ready, walk around the parking lot. Don't just sit!

My family really got into "The Walking Dead," when it came out. One thing I noticed, there were no fat walkers. They were all skinny … so keep walking.

Walk the dog?

I started out taking the dog with me on my walks. I figured she could use the exercise too. However, my dog thinks she is the Queen of the world. (Probably because that's how we treat her). So, in her regal roll, she feels it is necessary to bark at every dog, person or car that comes into sight. I tell her those big dogs could eat her for breakfast in one bite, but that doesn't seem to curtail her growls. Also, she has to stop and smell every single blade of grass in a square mile area.

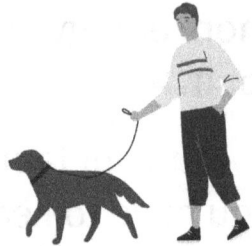

So, I find it difficult to keep a good pace when I bring her along. One day, she just decided she wasn't going any further and she laid down right there on the sidewalk! I had to carry her back home. Also, if she poops, I really don't want to carry that little bag of "blessings" for the entire trip!

There is a little old lady in my neighborhood who has a poodle type dog and she puts it in a stroller, bow and all, and walks it around the block.

There was a lady in my father's retirement community that would put her birdcage on her walker and take her bird for a walk.

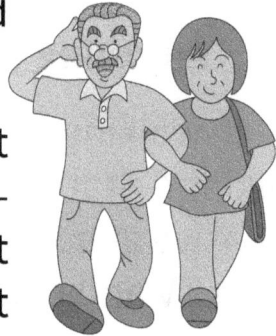

The bottom line is, if it doesn't slow your roll — take your dog, parakeet, pet alligator, whatever — just keep walking!

Don't get in a rut. Change it up. If you live near the beach, walk on the beach. If you are lucky enough to live in the mountains, there are thousands of hiking trails. Change it up, don't get in a rut.

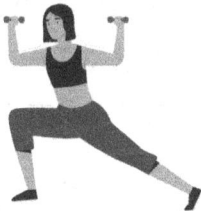

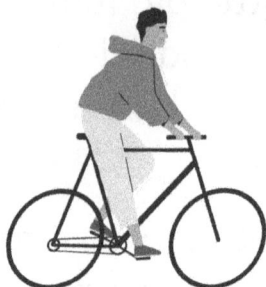

Anything that keeps you moving

If walking isn't your thing. How about biking? Stationary bikes can be quite inexpensive at a 2nd hand store. Sit it in front of your TV and pedal on.

There's an older couple in my neighborhood that ride their bikes every day. Most of your cities/towns have great biking trails. My husband and I used to ride bikes on the weekends years ago. It was great exercise. We ended up not doing it after our kids were born, but it was a great workout. My father used to ride his bike around the neighborhood when he was in his late 70s.

I will say this, you will probably never see me on a tandem bike. But I see tandem bikes all the time on the trails, so if that's your thing...pick a partner and pedal on.

There are hundreds of exercise videos on YouTube or Netflix or whatever may be available to you. You can find low impact aerobics videos that will do the trick. Start out small and work up. Most of these exercise routines require no equipment, just a little space. Again, get moving!

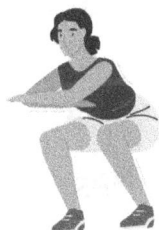

The best shape I have ever been in my life was when I joined a karate class. (I joined to meet guys). But, if that's your thing, do it. You will also have the added benefit of being able to defend yourself.

I think all of your YMCA's have water aerobic classes. I have done a few of these and they can give you a great workout!

Swimming is great! (And if you are like I was, it's a workout to just get in your bathing suit).

Join a country line dancing class. Get a work out with your HoeDown!

Whatever you choose, have a contingency plan. If it rains, I use my treadmill.

I have found that it is easier for me not to have to drive anywhere to do my exercise. It's too easy for me to come up with an excuse to not get up and get dressed and go.

Yes, it's great to have a walking or workout buddy. But, be determined. It also makes it easier if they don't come for you to say, well maybe I won't go either. Also, if you can carry on a conversation without getting winded while you are walking, you probably aren't walking fast enough. For aerobic exercise to be aerobic you need to be breathing heavily. I don't mean frantically panting, but oxygenating well!

The Oxford Language dictionary has the following definition for aerobic exercise.

"Relating to or denoting exercise that improves or is intended to improve the

efficiency of the body's cardiovascular system in absorbing and transporting oxygen."

You will find your pace improves over time. But, the goal is to get moving and keep a pace that will get your blood pumping!

I have joined several gyms over the years (again the goal was to meet guys). But, I found I wasn't consistent. It was easier to say "maybe not today". But, if that works for you do it! These days there are great opportunities out there that don't require contracts and are very reasonable. Most of them let you come and go whenever you want!

Do whatever it takes to help you enjoy your exercise times. Get a bluetooth head-set, put on your favorite oldies tunes and boogie on! Find some marching tunes. Listen to Sunday's sermon. Use this time to meditate or pray. I

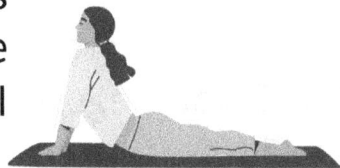

think I wrote most of this book in my head during my walks.

There is an old man that I see everyday when I walk. He is usually on the other side of the street. I can't hear what he is saying, but he walks and talks loudly. He is animated and moves his hands and arms all around. I've heard him sing as well. I don't know if he is praying or just talking to himself. But, he does seem to enjoy it.

My niece likes to run. As I said, I am not a runner. She also liked "The Walking Dead". She found a soundtrack of the growlers that she would listen to when she was running. She said when the growls got louder … she would run faster.

I also want to mention that I realize while I am writing this, there are some of you that can't even walk to your car without help. There are videos on the internet that you can use to exercise from your chair. If you can lift your legs, lift them. If you can move your arms, move them. Keep on moving ..

you want to keep and improve your range of motion and your endurance. Walk a little further, do a little more every day.

It has to become a habit. It has to become part of your routine. It needs to be such a part of your life, that you can't even imagine going back to a sedentary lifestyle.

At this point I want to say I am not giving you a number. Not a number of steps to hit every day, or a number of miles, or even a number of minutes. If you are overweight you are probably not eating correctly and/or not burning the calories that you consume. More than likely, you don't have any consistent exercise routine. You have to start where you are. Start small and keep moving. The goal is 5 lbs a month. You will not be able to do that if you don't do more physical activities to burn the calories.

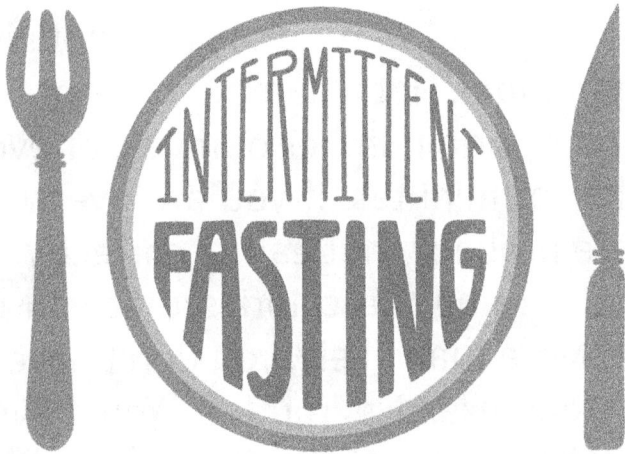

INTERMITTENT FASTING

Chapter 5

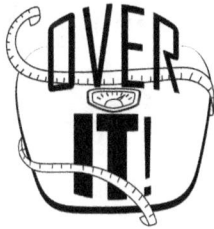

Fast a little

I don't eat anything past 5 o'clock at night. This helps me in several ways. First, I will eat less overall. I don't have a problem with the snacking urges if I have a hard and fast rule that I am done at 5:00pm.

I have it a little easier to cut it off early. My husband gets home at 4:00pm so if I cook, we can be done by 5:00pm. I also get up very early as I teach English to Chinese Children in the mornings. So, most days I am up by 5:00am. I go to bed most nights by 8:30pm.

If you don't get home from work until way after 5:00pm and don't go to bed until after 10:00pm, it may be a little more difficult to do this. My biggest suggestion is to make sure your evening meal is your ending meal for the day. It should also be your smallest meal of the day. And, quit eating long before you go to bed. You will find you eat less overall and you do not snack nearly as much.

Secondly, you will sleep better, you will have less acid reflux. Your body is in a rest mode when you sleep. If you eat late at night and then go to bed, you are not doing anything that requires energy. Your body takes any excess food and stores it. Where does it store it? That's right in your fat cells!

If you just can't possibly sit there or spend the evening without consuming something. Try a sugar free popsicle or some sugar free jello. Your body doesn't NEED the food...

You are just used to the endless snacks. We eat more out of habit than out of necessity.

I also use intermittent fasting to get back on track. If I have had a day where I have eaten too much, I will cut off eating at 2:00pm instead of 5:00pm.

There are benefits to having a fasting day where you just drink water or clear liquids. It can clean out toxins and help to improve your overall health.

In the past, I have had to deal with hypo-glycemia (low blood sugar) and was unable to fast. I would get dizzy and nauseous if I tried. I am better able to do it now. But, I still have a difficult time going all day without eating anything. I am able to cut off eating earlier however. That works for me.

There are benefits to fasting a day here or a day there. But, I would caution you not to try for much longer. At least until you know your overall metabolism is working efficiently. Smaller meals more often lets your body know it's not going to starve so it doesn't have to store food away.

Keep in mind people with anorexia may be skinny …. But they aren't healthy.

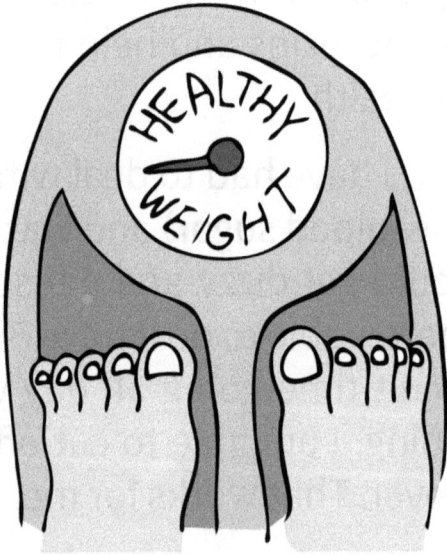

Chapter 6

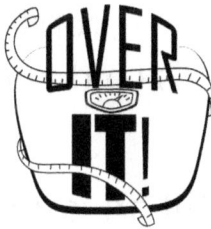

Water, Water Everywhere

You have heard this before. Your body needs water. Everything works better if you drink water. Especially if you work out .. you must stay hydrated.

10 glasses of water a day. --- more when you work out.

Now what's funny about this to me is, I have had no problems consuming 10 or more diet sodas a day. But, please oh please

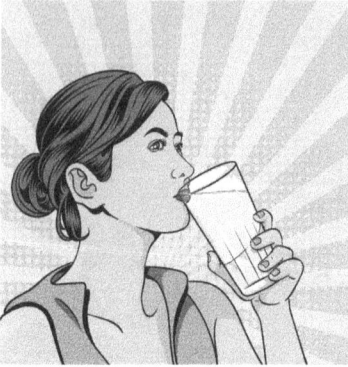

don't make me drink the water.

I still can't take straight water. It has to be cold, and it has to have some flavor drops. I can now drink it all day long if it's cold and has some kind of flavor.

Diet coke is still an issue with me. Years ago I used to say I would rather be fat than drink diet coke. That was true, until I got fat, and somewhere along the line I developed an addiction to it. I had a $20.00 a day coke habit (diet coke).

Of course, it's not good for you and it took its toll on my bladder. I was diagnosed with Interstitial Cystitis. Luckily, I was able to control it with diet. I cut out the diet coke and cut back on my coffee consumption and I haven't had issues.

I still find I want a diet coke a day. Sure, it's better than 16 a day, but I know it's not good for me.

Your energy drinks may sound good. But the caffeine is a jolt to your system and they are not good for you.

So what about your sports drinks? Keep in mind they were designed for "athletes" and most of my readers are not "athletes". They will replace your electrolytes but most are full of sugars.

Fruit juices are way too calorie rich and sugar rich as well.

The bottom line is, you can't replace the health benefits of water for staying well hydrated.

Try drinking a full 8 oz. of water before your meal. It will help to give you a "full" feeling and you will see you eat less.

Last Call for Alcohol

I thought this might be a good place to talk about alcohol.

Can I still have my wine and beer?

Well, wine is high in sugar. Beer, even low carb beer, is still full of empty calories. And certainly, one glass of wine or one low calorie/low carb beer every once in a while won't derail you.

If you drink 3-4 beers a day, or 3-4 glasses of wine or more a day, you will find it very difficult to lose weight. And, for the record, you aren't doing your liver any favors either.

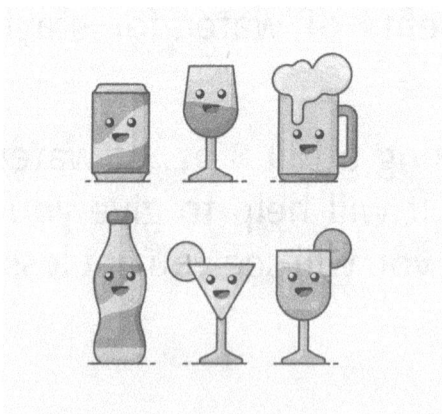

Chapter 7

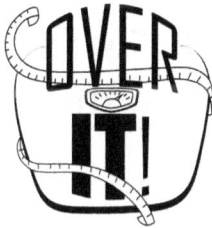

Journaling

It will help you to keep track and stay on track if you use a journal.

You can see your progress and your pitfalls.

Here are some sample entries.

January 2 —

I started the journey today. I am determined. I can do this. I will succeed. I ate well today, I made good choices and I was able to walk a little — not very far, not very fast — but a little. My weight is ___ and in one month's time it will be _____. Slow and steady.

January 15 —

I'm still on track. I've lost 3 whole pounds. I'm walking a little farther, and I do feel like I have more energy.

February 2 —

I did it ... 5 lbs down!! I'm still walking. I can make it all the way around the block!!! It's progress.

Today, I found a great recipe for a keto soup I want to try.

February 15 —

Every day I feel a little better. I can do this!

March 2 —

Wahoo! 10 lbs down!! I'm still wearing my fat clothes, but they feel a little looser.

I walked around the block today and I can tell I'm moving faster.

April 2 —

15 lbs. Down ! — I'm a quarter of the way to my goal for the year. I had a blouse that I could no longer wear. But it fit me today. Today was the first time someone asked me if I was losing weight!

April 15 —

It was a rough week, I had a cold and really didn't feel like working out. I did okay with eating, but it was hard to keep up with the exercising. It's okay.. I'm feeling better and will be back on track tomorrow. I may fast a little next week before I weigh in. But I realize I may have setbacks but I will continue going forward. No turning back!! No retreat!

May 2 —

My birthday! — We celebrated this weekend and I did have a piece of birthday cake.

(Before I would have eaten half the cake). I'm still making progress. 20 lbs. Down! I can do this!!

You get the idea. Rejoice with your victories, don't let the down days keep you down!! You can do this!

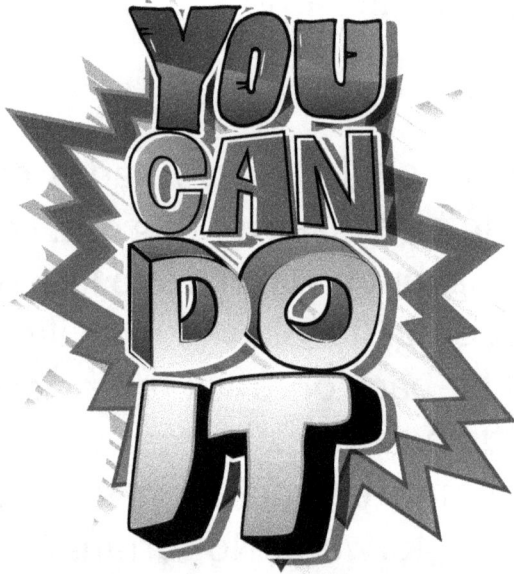

Chapter 8

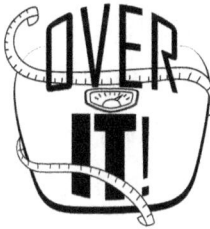

Plateaus and Pitfalls

I've done everything right and the scale is not budging. It has been stuck on the same number for days!

Many years ago, I came down with a sinus infection that literally lasted for months. Three rounds of antibiotics later, and I was still feeling horrible and still running a fever. Finally, I started to get better, feel better and have more energy. But, I was still running a low grade fever. After a couple of weeks of that I talked with my mother, who was a nurse. I told her I was feeling fine, but still running a low grade fever. Here was her response…. "If you are feeling fine, quit taking your temperature!"

So, if you are doing everything right, trust me eventually the scale will move. There were a few months where I didn't meet my goal weight on the 2nd. One month it wasn't until the 10th of the month that I finally hit the 5lb goal! Just keep on keeping on … Stay off the scale!!

My dad had an older car and the "check engine" light came on. He took it to the mechanic and the mechanic checked it all out and told him everything was fine. The car was running right and he didn't have any issues. But, that darned "check engine" light was burning brightly and kept bugging my dad. So finally, he got some black electrical tape and put it over the light… problem solved!

Maybe we need some of the black tape for our scales!

Make the plan, stick to the plan and eventually the weight will come off, the energy will get better and your clothes will get looser. Keep going!

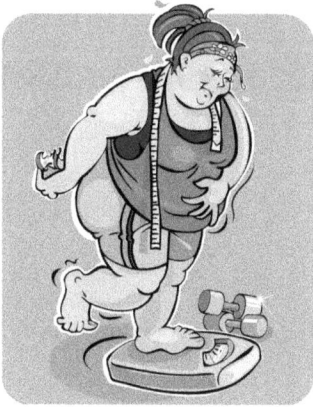

Sometimes, the scale stays stuck, because you are constipated. I find that if I eat a lot of cheese, or maybe after a big meat day, I get a little backed up. If this is TMI for you, read on. ... But, I have found that more roughage and more fruits will keep me regular.

Also, the Smooth Move tea at the grocery store does the trick. However, I caution you to not grow to rely on laxatives or laxative products. This is not how your body was designed, and it will become used to them.

And, you may find you can't "go" without them. (pun intended).

So, if you find yourself at your end-of-the month weigh in and you haven't met your 5 lb goal for the month, here are some suggestions to help get you over the hump!

1. Have a fast day

2. Stop eating at 2pm today instead of the usual after dinner time.

3. Have an all liquids day … (nothing but protein shakes today).

4. Maybe do two exercise routines in a day.

5. But most importantly, don't get discouraged and don't quit. It's basic physics. If you eat less and exercise more eventually the weight will come off!

Get up right now, go to the mirror, look straight in the mirror, point to yourself, look yourself right in the eyes and say …

Don't you dare quit!!!

One of my favorite preachers has a saying.

"I may not be where I need to be, but thank God I'm not where I used to be. I am OK and I am on my way!

What is fun about the plateaus is, eventually they stop and the scale moves. It's always fun when you see it jump. And, there is much more chance of that if you only weigh twice a month! The scale can be your friend, but it can also become your enemy. Don't let it be your enemy!

you got this

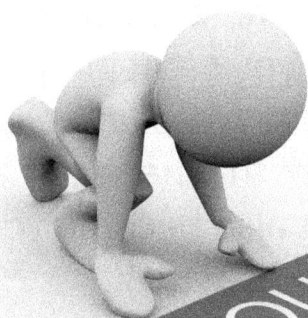
ARE YOU READY?

Chapter 9

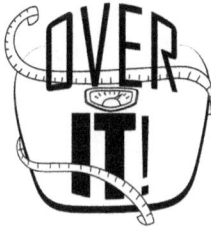

Getting started tips

It will help if you go on some type of cleanse to begin your journey.

I do recommend the cabbage soup diet. It's a good cleansing plan for a full week and will help to cleanse your body of some toxins, help to alleviate your cravings, and get you moving toward your low carb lifestyle.

I like it because you can eat as much cabbage soup as you like and it actually tastes good.

I got the following directly from their website. www.healthline.com/nutrition/the-cabbage-soup-diet#basic-steps

The Cabbage Soup Recipe

Ingredients:

- 2 large onions
- 2 green peppers
- 2 cans of tomatoes
- 1 bunch of celery
- 1 head of cabbage
- 3 carrots
- 1 package of mushrooms
- 1–2 bouillon cubes (optional)
- 6–8 cups of water or vegetable cocktail, such as V8

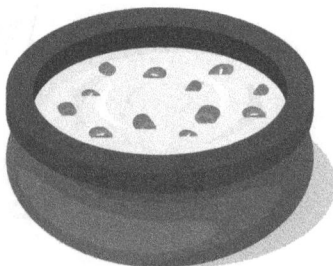

Directions:

1. Chop all vegetables into cubes.

2. In a large stock pot, sauté onions in a small amount of oil.

3. Then add the remaining vegetables and cover with water or vegetable cocktail and add bouillon cubes or other seasonings, if desired.

4. Bring to a boil, then reduce to medium heat. Let simmer until vegetables are tender, about 30–45 minutes.

You may season the soup with salt, pepper, hot sauce, herbs or spices. You may also add other non-starchy vegetables such as spinach or green beans.

Every day, you should eat as much cabbage soup as you want — at least for several meals.

Rules of the Diet

You are allowed to eat 1–2 other low-calorie foods daily in addition to the soup.

However, it is important not to make any other substitutions and to drink only water or other calorie-free beverages, such as unsweetened tea.

A daily multivitamin is often recommended because the diet may be low in certain nutrients.

These are the rules for each day of the Cabbage Soup Diet.

- **Day 1**: Unlimited cabbage soup and fruit, but no bananas.

- **Day 2**: Only soup and vegetables. Focus on raw or cooked leafy greens. Avoid peas, corn and beans. You may also have one baked potato with butter or oil.

- **Day 3**: As many fruits and vegetables as you can eat, in addition to the soup. However, no baked potato and no bananas.

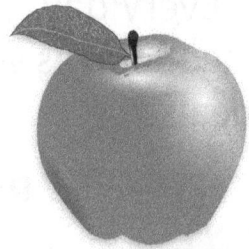

- **Day 4**: Unlimited bananas, skim milk and cabbage soup.

- **Day 5**: You are allowed 10–20 ounces (280–567 grams) of beef, which you may substitute for chicken or fish. You may also have up to six fresh tomatoes. Drink at least 6–8 glasses of water.

- **Day 6**: Soup, beef and vegetables. You may substitute the beef for broiled fish if you did not do so the day prior. Focus on leafy greens. No baked potato.

- **Day 7**: You may have vegetables, brown rice and unlimited fruit juice — but no added sugar.

You should not continue the diet for more than seven days at a time. However, you may repeat the diet as long as you wait at least two weeks before starting it again.

I like this one week diet cleanse. I think it's a good way to get started. However, it's not the only way.

Maybe do a clear liquids fast for a day.

There are certainly other cleansing routines. Remember, these are not forever suggestions. However, I do recommend using one of them, just to get you started. This cleanse will help give you a good jump-start!

Plan Ahead

Place your workout clothes or shoes out. If you wait until you get to work to walk, be sure and put your walking shoes on and carry your dress shoes with you.

Pack a lunch and some snacks the night before so all you have to do is grab it and run.

If you want to use a workout video … find one you like and queue it up. Get everything you need ready.

Get your water bottles/drinking mugs ready.

Make sure you have your step counter ready.

I have a rechargeable fan that I use. I make sure when I come home from my walk, it is plugged in and re-charging ready for my next walk. My hat is always in the same place.

Check the weather, if you know it's going to rain make sure you are ready for your alternate workout whatever that is.

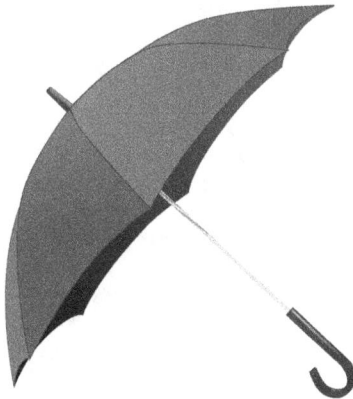

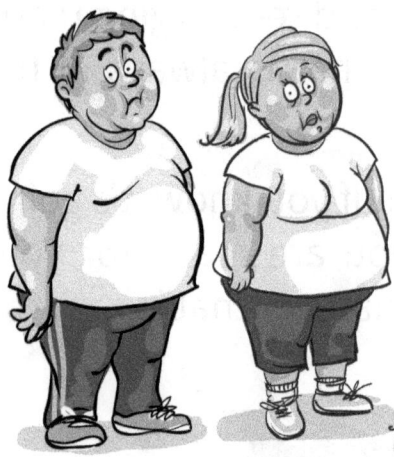

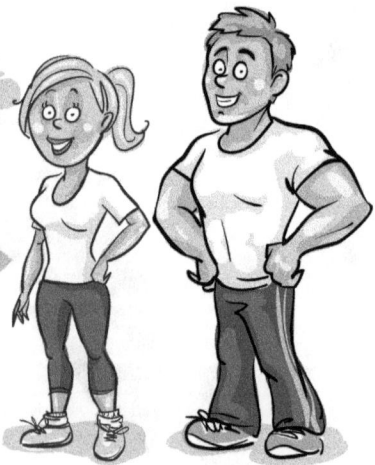

Chapter 10

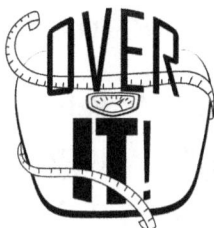

I did it! What now?

Congratulations! You have succeeded! It is such a wonderful feeling to have set a goal and met your goal! Especially a long term goal like this one!

I know you are feeling good, and looking good!

So, the absolute most important thing now is ... you have to keep it off! You are healthier now! Stay that way!

I have decided I am NEVER going back. I like being skinny again. I like wearing skinny clothes and I like having more energy. I like staying active and feeling better.

So, here's the deal. Yes, you can eat a little more because you are now in a sustaining mode and don't have to be in a losing mode.

BUT, if you add back in the carbs and the sugars your weight will go up! And, because of the way our bodies metabolize those sugars and the carbs, your weight will go back up very quickly.

Remember, the cravings will return when your blood sugar fluctuates.

I still maintain a very low carb diet. But here's the good news, I do occasionally allow myself the piece of cake or cookie or chocolate. And, I actually will weigh myself more often to make sure I haven't started putting back on the weight. If I have gained a little, I might fast a little. I may have a cleansing day to assure I'm staying where I want to be.

Walking and exercising need to be "forever changes". The more active you remain, the more healthy you will be long-term. Activity will help to stave off osteoporosis, heart issues, and high blood pressure.

When my father was aging, he lived in an assisted living facility. There was a lady that lived there that was in her late 80s, but still walked 5 miles a day. She was only a resident there because her husband needed the care. After he passed, she found an apartment and moved out and she remained independent. She would come back and visit, she was still walking 5 miles a day.

Your mind will stay alert longer. Your heart will stay stronger longer.

This is my long term goal. I want to stay healthy, and stay independent for

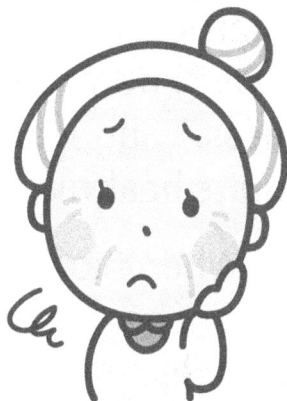

the rest of my life. I do not want to become a burden to my family.

My paternal grandmother lived long and stayed healthy. When it was her time to go, she told my aunt. "I'm going to go see Mr. Guess today." (that's what she called her late husband). She then went into her room and laid on her bed and died. She wasn't sick, she wasn't feeble, she just left and went to Heaven.

I had a great aunt who waited until she was 98 before she checked herself into an Assisted Living Community. She lived to be over 100 and her mind was still intact. The local paper interviewed her on her 100th birthday and they asked her why she never married. Her response to the young reporter was "I don't think that is any of your business." She was sweet and sassy, and still quite healthy.

When I look at my future, I want it to be one of health and happiness. Not a future of sickness, disease and nursing homes.

My father developed Parkinsons in his mid-70's. Thankfully it was relatively slow progressing. But, eventually he needed round the clock care. Unfortunately, we didn't have the financial means to afford in-home care and we could not care for him ourselves. We all worked and even then, didn't have the strength to be able to lift him. He needed meds, and our only alternative was a long-term care facility. We made sure one of us was able to visit him every day. But, it was still a very difficult time for us.

It was a terribly depressing place. Many people were there with debilitating diseases. Diabetics, that had to have limbs amputated. People bound to wheelchairs, people on oxygen. I do not want to end up like that!

I believe for most of us, a healthy long life can be a choice. It will be

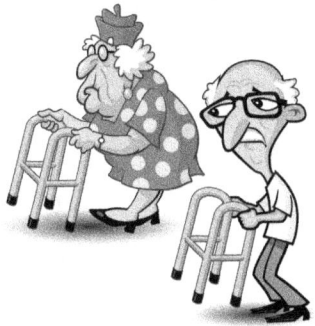

determined in a very large part by your diet and your activity level.

Keep it up!

You did it … You achieved Your goal. Stay healthy!

I want to hear from you. Please, send me your success stories and your questions.

www.Over50Overweightandoverit.com

Go get some new clothes!!! Enjoy yourself! Celebrate!

Yes! you did it!

This may be helpful to you. I have included the web addresses where I have copied from.

https://docs.google.com/ document/d/1yp8RsnZLafEard6mDV-BqVBa_N4x7zdbBdVS6MshAPA/ edit#

The glycemic index is a system of assigning a number to carbohydrate-containing foods according to how much each food increases blood sugar. The glycemic index itself is not a diet plan but one of various tools — such as calorie counting or carbohydrate counting — for guiding food choices

https://docs.google.com/ document/d/1yp8RsnZLafEard6mDV-BqVBa_N4x7zdbBdVS6MshAPA/ edit#

Glycemic Index

Low GI (<55), Medium GI (56-69) and High GI (70>)

Grains / Starchs		Vegetables		Fruits		Dairy		Proteins	
Rice Bran	27	Asparagus	15	Grapefruit	25	Low-Fat Yogurt	14	Peanuts	21
Bran Cereal	42	Broccoli	15	Apple	38	Plain Yogurt	14	Beans, Dried	40
Spaghetti	42	Celery	15	Peach	42	Whole Milk	27	Lentils	41
Corn, sweet	54	Cucumber	15	Orange	44	Soy Milk	30	Kidney Beans	41
Wild Rice	57	Lettuce	15	Grape	46	Fat-Free Milk	32	Split Peas	45
Sweet Potatoes	61	Peppers	15	Banana	54	Skim Milk	32	Lima Beans	46
White Rice	64	Spinach	15	Mango	56	Chocolate Milk	35	Chickpeas	47
Cous Cous	65	Tomatoes	15	Pineapple	66	Fruit Yogurt	36	Pinto Beans	55
Whole Wheat Bread	71	Chickpeas	33	Watermelon	72	Ice Cream	61	Black-Eyed Beans	59
Muesli	80	Cooked Carrots	39						
Baked Potatoes	85								
Oatmeal	87								
Taco Shells	97								
White Bread	100								

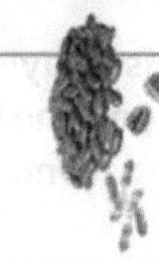

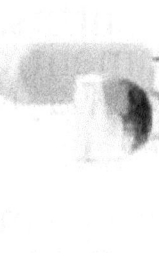

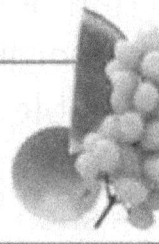

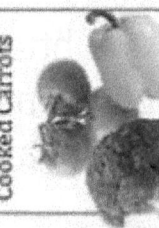